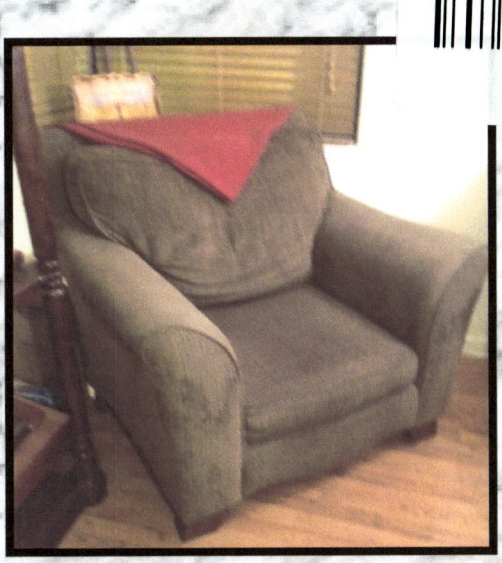

The Complete

Easychair Workout

Program (+)

A whole-body workout routine you can do

for your first _100 years,_ without having to

leave the comfort of your _easychair!_

The Complete Easychair Workout Program   **Dr. Rick Boatright**

This book is dedicated to all conscien-
tious objectors who, like me, resist
getting up out of that perfectly nice,
comfy, easychair for such dreaded
self-torture as "exercise," ... but who,
deep down, know they should be
exercising on a regular basis for a
long and health life!

Table of contents

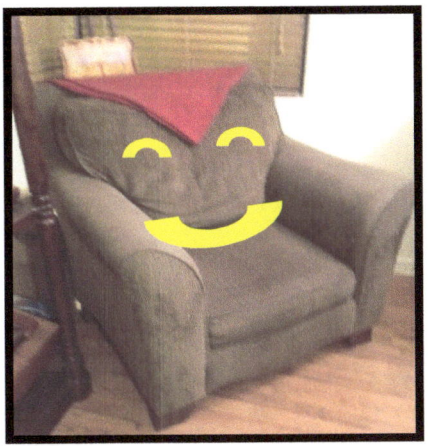

Chapter 1: Your Easychair Is Your Friend!

Well past retirement age and in my late 60's, I still work my tail off! I maintain one office in Phoenix, Arizona and another one 190 miles away in a small mountain town called Show Low. I work 2 1/2 days a week in Phoenix and one day in Show Low … seeing human patients.

I drive almost 400 miles a week on this commute alone. But I also have a side practice working on horses. It's common for me to drive an extra 200 miles on a horse day. Needless to say, I'm busier than a cat trying to cover up a mess on a marble floor!

But my real love is writing. So "in my spare time," I write … books, newsletters, web sites, e-books, video scripts and more. (See my writer's web site at **www.readem.net**.)

Plus I'm active with church leadership responsibilities in Arizona.

For an old guy, I'm fairly busy. My "free time" is _**precious**_ to me. I have this persistent resistance to "exercising" … just moving around for the sake of moving around … while I could be getting other things done … or resting!

One morning I was sitting in my easychair for ten minutes, waiting for my lovely wife, Linda, to finish getting ready for work and it hit me in the face like a three-ton pillow!

I don't HAVE TO get up, dance around, lift weights, or any of that traditional exercise stuff. I can get a ***good*** workout sitting right here in that big, comfy, overstuffed chair doing "isometric" exercises!

With isometric exercises, we apply effort against resistance, but without moving the joints and muscles.

Whether I want to work my thighs to help me with leg strength and balance, work my arms, strengthen my back or tone my tummy, I can work all the muscle groups I need to work sitting right there.

And so can you!

Will it make you look like Arnold Schwarzenegger or a fashion model? Probably not, unless, of course, you already do, even though this is similar to the exercises that Charles Atlas implemented to produce his chiseled physique.

This exercise program is PRACTICAL. It's perfect for lazy people like me, and people who DO want to do something real and tangible to stay in shape. That way when we're 100, we can still play golf or go out to dinner with family or live more independently than our surviving peers.

You can do these exercises if you're disabled. You can do them if you can't stand up. You can do them if you have a hard time keeping your balance. You can exercise if you have limiting injuries. ***You'll be sitting in your easychair***! If any particular exercise hurts, just say "OK," skip that one and go on the next.

How vigorously you do this exercise program is your choice. The more committed you get, the more benefits you'll receive. But even a half-hearted effort done _regularly_ makes a huge difference over a period of months or years.

I don't know about you, but if I'm going to live to 102 (and I plan to do just that) I want to do everything I can to make sure I can walk, get around on my own, and have the strength and endurance I need to truly enjoy my life as I get there.

Don't want to get up and exercise? You DON'T HAVE TO! You can do it sitting right there in your easychair.

How do I know?

I mentioned before that I'm a doctor ... a doctor of chiropractic. I know how every bone in the body moves and which muscles attach to each one of them. I've been at it so long, I have peers in my profession today who were born AFTER I got my license to practice.

Chiropractors have a particularly intricate understanding of how specific exercises can benefit particular body areas.

I've put that understanding to practical application in this book to help you _achieve your own goals_.

I've written this book thinking about middle-agers and older; however, it will help young adults improve their physical conditioning too.

You see, the hardest part about any exercise program is convincing ourselves to DO it. Most of us fall to the wayside because:

- We don't want to get dressed and go to the gym.

- We don't want to go outside when it's raining, or too hot, or too cold, or too snowy, or too dry ...

- We've hung too many clothes on the treadmill or stair stepper.

- We have too hard a time getting up from the rowing machine.

- It's Sunday.

- It's a holiday.

- It's a workday.

- It's our day off.

- We simply don't want to get up out of that comfy, overstuffed easy-chair to do ANYTHING!

But with this program, once you learn it and practice it a few times, you'll have a tool you can keep in your fitness arsenal … and use at your *leisure* … for the rest of your life. Ideally, you'll set a schedule to do the program regularly.

But even if you don't and one afternoon you're sitting in front of the tube thinking, "Gosh, I just have to start doing SOMETHING to get more exercise," you won't even have to get up out of that chair! You can start right where you are. In fact, you won't even have to sit up straight! You can *slouch* and get right into it!

So without further preamble, let's jump right in. Go to the next page and let's get started!

* * *

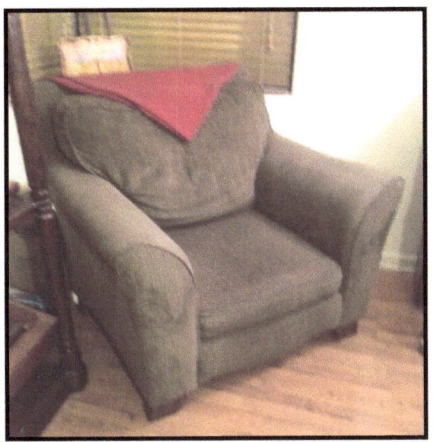

Chapter 2: The Ideal Chair

You probably thought that when I said you'd be exercising in an "easychair," I was really talking about sitting in a hard-seated, straight-backed chair.

Not on your life!

It doesn't have to be pretty. It just needs to be a deep, comfy, cushy kind of real easychair. In fact, anything less is going to lack some specific features you'll need for accomplishing the exercises I'll be describing.

Let me start with a full description of the ideal easychair for doing these exercises. *(Use this description as your argument to go out and buy one if you need to!)* It's an investment in a piece of "exercise equipment" that will give you many happy returns, even when you're not using it for its exercise qualities!

1) The chair should be low so that your feet easily rest on the floor when you're slouching. This ensures that you can do your leg and tummy exercises with the greatest ease and comfort, plus the most efficiency.

1) The back of the chair should be far enough back that you'll have to slouch to let your knees bend at the front end of the seat cushion. This helps maximize the effectiveness of your tummy exercises.

2) You'll want tall arms at the sides. You should NOT be able to let your elbows rest at your sides and still have them above the tops of the armrests. Ideally, your elbows should come up to—or near—shoulder height when you slouch. With tall arms on your easychair, you'll have the "equipment" you'll need for your arm, back and shoulder exercises.

If you don't already have a chair like this, now you have the perfect excuse to go out and get one! Happy shopping!

* * *

Back is far enough from the front of the seat cushion

High arms

Low front

Cushy and Comfy!

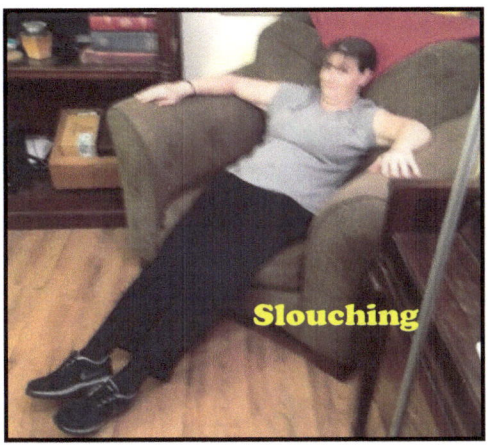

Slouching

Chapter 3: Assume the Position!

Throughout the book, I'll refer to "assuming the position." This position forms the basic slouch from which you start the majority of exercises.

Here's how that goes. And here's how that looks.

Sit in the center of the seat cushion so that your low back is NOT in contact with the back cushion. Make sure your knees are off the front end of the seat cushion and your feet are resting out in front of you on the floor.

Lean back so your upper back is resting against the back of the chair. This should place you into a nice, comfortable, slouching position.

Place your arms flat on top of the chair arms.

As crazy as it may seem, you'll be in the perfect posture to do this simple but powerful exercise program.

# # #

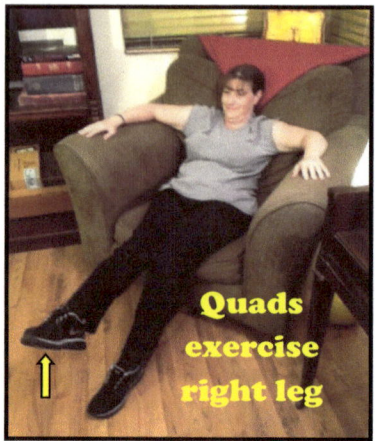

Quads exercise right leg

Chapter 4: Lower Extremities

Sometimes we just have to start with something easy and work up the motivation to get more aggressive. With this program, interestingly enough, we start with what SEEMS to be the least effort. But we'll be working on the biggest muscle groups in the body. When we use these babies, we burn the most calories!

The best part is that we don't have to climb stairs or walk for miles to work these muscles. Of course, I'm referring to the thigh muscles.

There are two major muscle groups in the thighs: the quadriceps … or "quads" for short ... and the hamstrings.

The Quads Exercise: The quads are the large muscles on the _fronts_ of your thighs. They're the muscles that straighten your legs at the knees, and, to a much lesser degree, bend your legs at the hips.

The first exercise we'll do is contracting the quads. So, first, _assume the position_. Straighten your left leg straight out in front of you so that your knee is no longer bent and your foot is about 6 to 8 inches off the floor. Hold the leg and foot straight out in front of you for a count of ten. Then, _slowly_ lower it back to the floor. Wasn't that easy? Then repeat the exercise with the right leg.

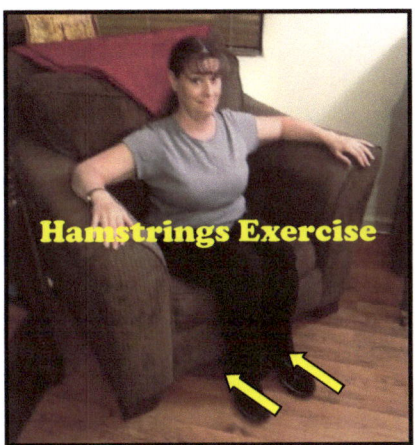

I like to have people set a goal of twenty of these on each side in a set. If you're not in good enough condition to do that, do as many as you can and then go on to the next exercise.

If this doesn't seem to challenge you at all, do more. The same will be true for every exercise in this book. So I'll state my easy recommendation and you can adjust it as you like.

Like all exercises in this book, if it hurts—STOP!

The Hamstrings Exercise: The thing about working any muscle group is that you need to achieve balance. So the next exercise is to work the muscle group on the opposite side of your thighs—the hamstrings. These are long, slender muscles on the *backs* of your thighs. They're responsible for bending your knees and they assist in bringing you to a standing position when you're bent at the waist. *(But don't panic! We're not going to do toe touches!)*

We'll work these muscles in a sitting position in your easychair by bending your legs at the knees … against resistance.

In our daily activities, most of us work our quads … the ones on the front … much more often than our hamstrings . So most of us have *under-developed* hamstrings when compared to our quads.

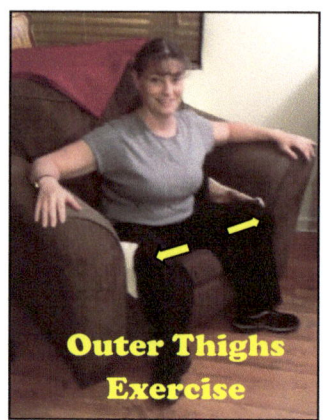

Therefore we're going to work the hamstrings a little harder and use resistance to build their strength better.

For the hamstrings exercise, sit a little straighter. Scoot back in the chair so that the backs of your calves are touching the front of the chair.

Then press the backs of both calves and feet into the front of the chair. Use as much pressure as you feel comfortable exerting. Hold it for ten seconds.

Do ten of these in a set.

As you gain strength over time, pressing harder will increase your strength even more. Some say that building strength in your hamstrings contributes to helping you stay stable on your feet.

The Outer Thigh Exercise: Do this exercise, sitting straight up in the chair, or slouching in "the position." If your easychair has arms that are particularly far apart, you may need to get some firm cushions or pillows to place between the arms of the chair and the outsides of your thighs. (See the illustration above.)

This exercise involves pressing your thighs and knees outward against

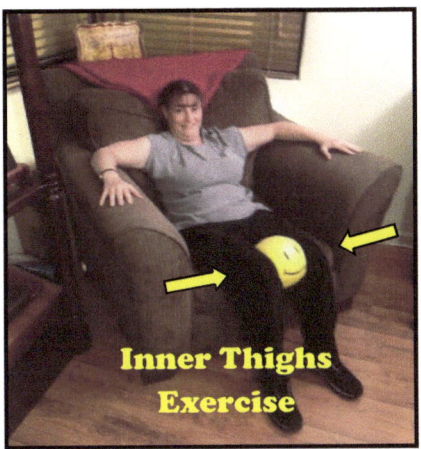

Inner Thighs
Exercise

the resistance of the arms of your easychair.

If you have hip socket issues, please be cautious about doing this one. If you experience the slightest bit of sharp pain in your groin or outer, upper thighs, stop immediately and go to the next exercise. You may also want to consult an Activator chiropractor (www.activator.com) or an orthopedic doctor to evaluate your hip sockets.

Otherwise, press outward with both knees at the same time and hold for ten seconds. The amount of pressure you exert is up to you. More pressure offers greater benefits but you don't have to conquer the world in an afternoon.

For safety and good habit-building, I recommend starting out with the ridiculously easy and working your way up very slowly.

Shoot for ten repetitions in a set.

Inner Thighs Exercise: Next, move on to the Inner Thighs Exercise. For this one, use the full slouch position. Get really comfortable.

Again, you judge how much pressure your use, remembering that the more pressure you exert, the more benefit you gain. Our muscles always adapt to the amount of exertion we put them through on a

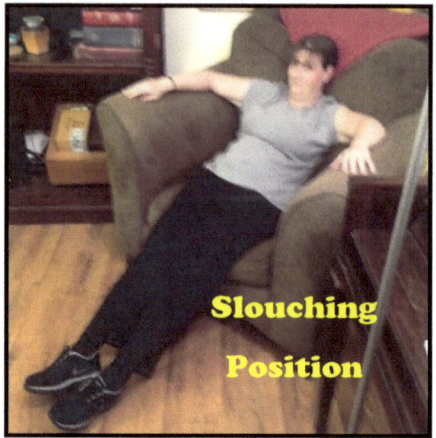

regular basis. That's how exercise builds strength over time.

To exercise your inner thighs, simply press your knees together quite firmly and hold for ten seconds. Then repeat ten times. If you prefer, you can place a cushion or a ball between your knees and press into the ball like I do. (See illustration on previous page.) Simple, huh!

Let me explain WHY muscles get stronger when we use them. It's also the reason why we have more energy 24/7/365 when we exercise on a regular basis.

Inside our cells are little components called "organelles." There are several kinds of organelles in cells. One group is called "mitochondria." These little "factories" inside our cells turn our food into useable energy.

When we exercise on a regular basis, it stimulates the mitochondria in our muscle cells to reproduce faster. They get more abundant. It's our body's way of trying to keep up with anticipated energy demands.

The more we exercise, the stronger we get and the more energy we have … all the time. It sounds backward, but that's how the body works.

By now, we've done a good job exercising all of the muscle groups in the thighs.

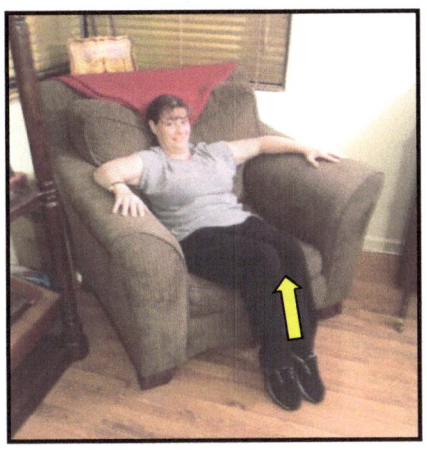

Calf Raise Exercise

So lets go down to the calves.

Calf Raise Exercises: Assume the slouching position again for this one. Place your hands on the arm rests. Raise both heels up as far as you can by straightening out your ankles. Your toes stay on the floor. Hold this straight for ten seconds and repeat. The goal here? … Do both sides _twenty_ times. (Otherwise it's just _too_ easy.)

If you want to add more resistance, lean forward, pressing down with your upper body weight resting on your hands or elbows, placed on your knees.

By doing the easychair leg exercises regularly and pushing yourself just a little; over time, you'll gain more strength to walk with the kids and grandkids, to play golf if you like, to be steadier on your feet and safer from stumbles and falls around home. Plus, those calves will be looking fine!

You'll gain more energy, more stamina and be in a generally better mood.

But working the legs is just the beginning. We want to help you get as fit as possible from your toes all the way up.

# # #

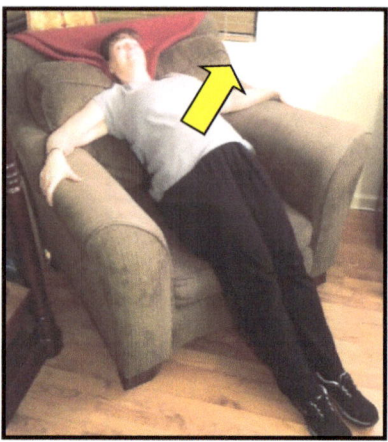

Chapter Five: The Torso

Staying with larger muscle groups and working our way down to smaller muscle groups, let's take up working on our low back muscles. The stronger we can get those babies, the better we'll be able to fight off that chronic low back pain. It won't take the place of your chiropractor's adjustments; but it will usually make the doctor's work hold better and resolve faster. *Be sure to check with your doc before you do this one if you have chronic low back pain.*

Low Back Exercise: For this important exercise, *assume the position.* Full slouch. Put your feet in front of you as far as you can with the backs of your heels on the floor.

Then lift and straighten our body to make it rigid, supporting your weight on two points … the backs of your thighs, just above your knees, and the backs of your shoulders. Hold it for 3 to 5 seconds to start. Over time, work your way up to 10 to 20 seconds. Repeat ten times.

You'll have to contract your low back (and buttock) muscles to accomplish this. You'll get a double benefit from this one. It also replaces the toe touches we all shy away from so ardently.

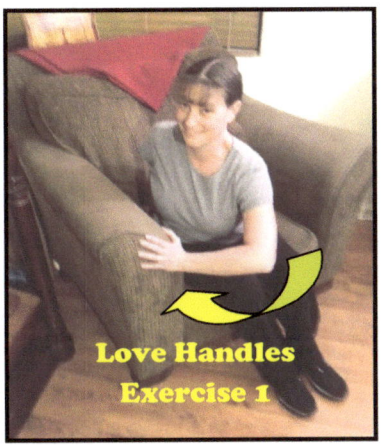

You won't even have to stand. And just think! You can exercise your **_bottom_** without having to get out of the chair! How cool is that?!

Want to work on those "love handles?" They're next!

The Love Handles Exercise: Unfortunately, we can't start this one in the slouch position. But who cares, if we can attack those puffy, little, muffin - top love handles?

Position yourself near the front of the seat cushion sitting straight up. Reach around your body with your left hand and grasp the inside-front of the right chair arm. Then use the muscles at your waist to twist your body, pressing against the resistance of the hand that's holding the chair's arm. (See the illustration.)

Hold the resistance for ten seconds. Then repeat the exercise on the other side. Aim for ten times on each side.

It's a small price to pay for trimming down those ugly, little, side bulges. And it's a whole lot more fun than holding weights and doing side bends in front of a mirror and a room full of people at the gym!

The next, most logical muscle group would be the tummy muscles

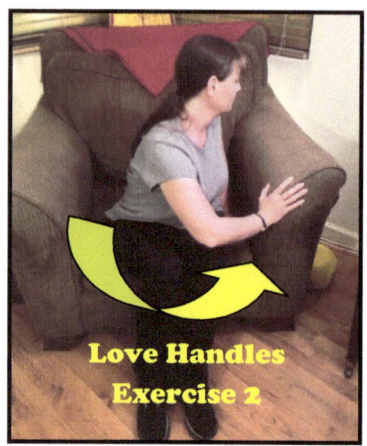

… building that six-pack. (Just kidding.) We **_will_** be strengthening and trimming that mid section however, but not just yet. Statistically, working the tummy muscles works best when it's done at the end of your workout. So we'll come back to those.

The next group of large muscles are those in the upper back.

Please keep in mind that throughout this entire protocol so far, you've never once had to leave your easychair!

Now, let's put some work into two different upper back muscle groups.

Push-Back Exercise: If you were in the gym, you'd have to pull on cables or bend over a bench with weights or sit in a rowing machine to do this one. But **_you_** can stay right there in your easychair!

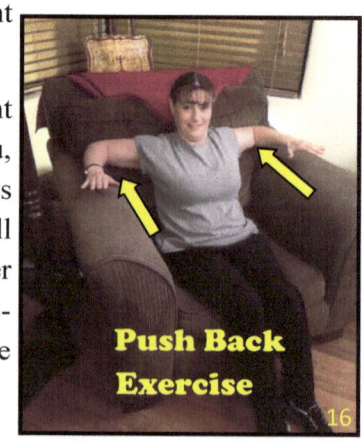

Raise your elbows to shoulder height with your hands out in front of you, palms down. Simply push your elbows back into the back cushion. Really pull with the muscles between your shoulder blades. Hold the pressure for ten seconds, then relax. Train yourself to do the exercise for ten repetitions in a set.

16

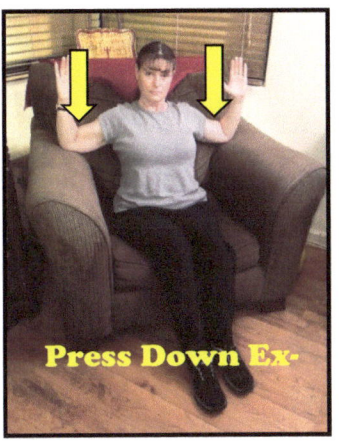

Press Down Ex-

Press-Down Exercises: Place your elbows straight out to your sides, on the tops of the chair arms with your hands straight up, palms forward.

Press your elbows downward into both chair arms at the same time and hold for ten seconds.

Ten repetitions is the goal.

Strengthening your upper back with these last two exercises can help people get over some of that persistent mid back and shoulder achiness that's so nagging at the end of the day. For some, it even reduces the frequency and severity of tension headaches.

Surprisingly, so can chest exercises.

Chest exercises: This is actually just an old Charles Atlas exercise. It has little to do with the chair. Simply make yourself comfortable. It's a three-part exercise to make sure you get all three parts of your chest muscles.

♦ First put your hands together at shoulder level with our fingers pointing straight forward. Press your hands together, hard. Hold it for ten seconds. Repeat ten times.

♦ Do a second set exactly the same, except with your hands down at

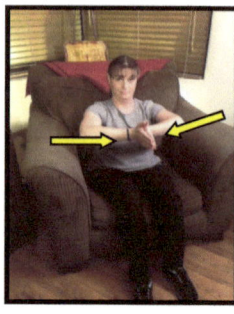 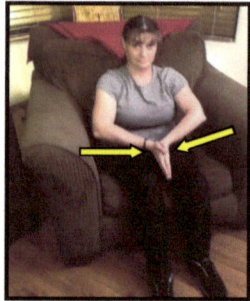 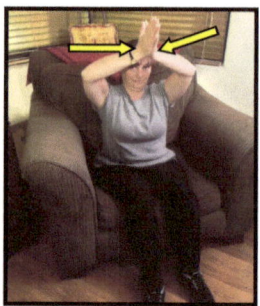

tummy level.

♦ Finally, do a third set with your hands at face level.

The harder you press your hands together, the more you strengthen your chest muscles. How hard you press is up to you.

Just be cautious if you have wrist challenges like carpal tunnel syndrome.

One of the most useful exercises you can do in an easychair for whole body health is one that repositions your head up over your shoulders where it's supposed to be.

More than 90 percent of Americans carry their heads at least one inch forward of the optimal position. I've seen people who carry their heads four, five or even six inches forward.

We spend 12 years going to school, studying with our heads down. Many of us spend several more years going to college with our heads down. Then we go to work and keep our heads down toward our desk papers and go home to read the paper in our laps. Not to mention the time we spend on our smart phones!

It's no wonder the muscles in the backs of our necks elongate and waste away and the ones in front get short and weak. So our next exercise is going to address this.

# # #

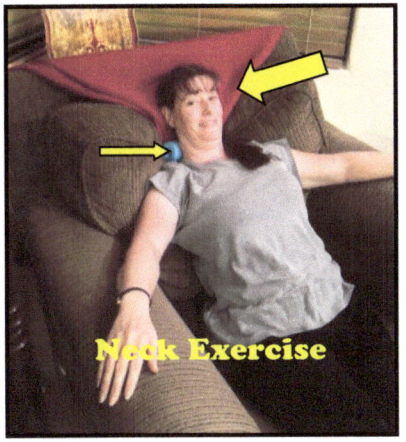

Neck Exercise

Chapter 6:

Neck and Upper Extremities

Neck Exercise: This exercise can change your entire body posture, give you more balance and even decrease low back pain in some instances.

Assume the position. Then press your head backward into the back of the chair. Hold it for ten seconds and repeat ten times.

It can work even better if you cut a 7-inch piece of a swimming pool noodle and place it behind your neck during the exercise.

I recommend the pool noodle for nearly every patient who comes into my office with neck pain!

Would you like to address the backs of your upper arms? Let's do that next.

Triceps Exercise: Sit comfortably in your easychair. Place your arms and hands against the chair arms. Keeping your elbows in contact with the arms of the chair, press into the chair arms, hard, with your forearms and hands. Hold it for 10 seconds

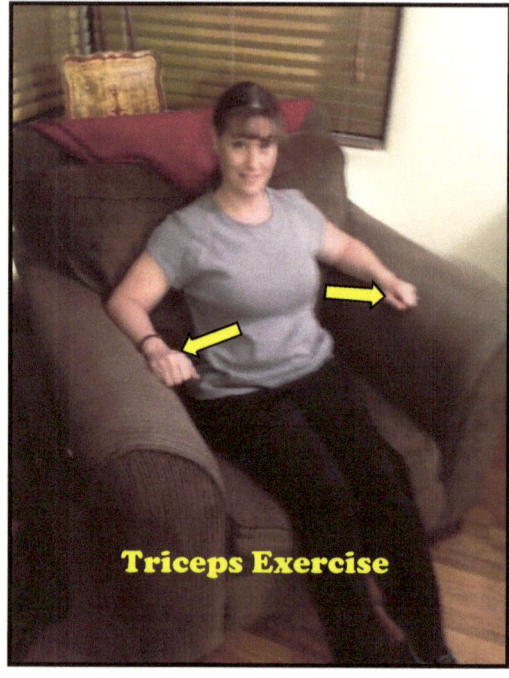

Triceps Exercise

and repeat ten times.

This works the muscles on the backs of your arms. It may not shrink the _skin_ on the backs of your arms, but it _will_ tone the muscles there.

You'll work the fronts of your upper arms … your biceps … by using the arms of the chair too.

Biceps Exercise: To contract your biceps against resistance, hang your arms over the sides of the chair's arms. Press into the outsides of the chair with both hands. Hold for ten seconds and repeat ten times. This exercises replaces the "dumbbell curls" you'd have to be pumping out at the gym for your upper arms!

Shoulder Exercise: Exercise your shoulders while you're here too. Place your elbows close to your body INSIDE the arms of the chair.

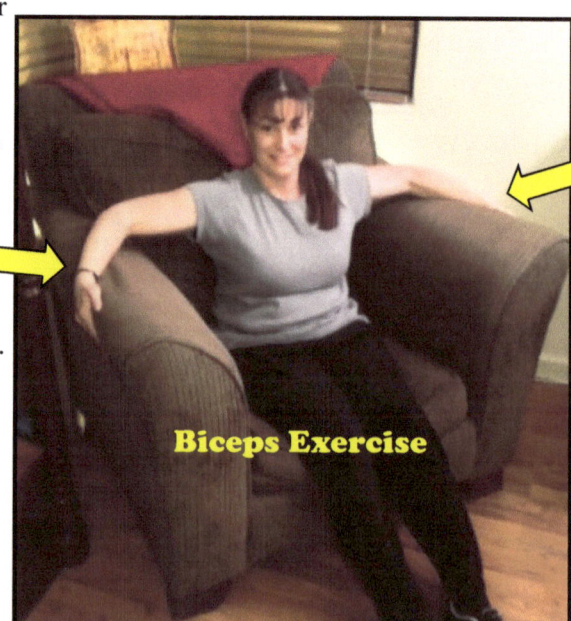

Biceps Exercise

20

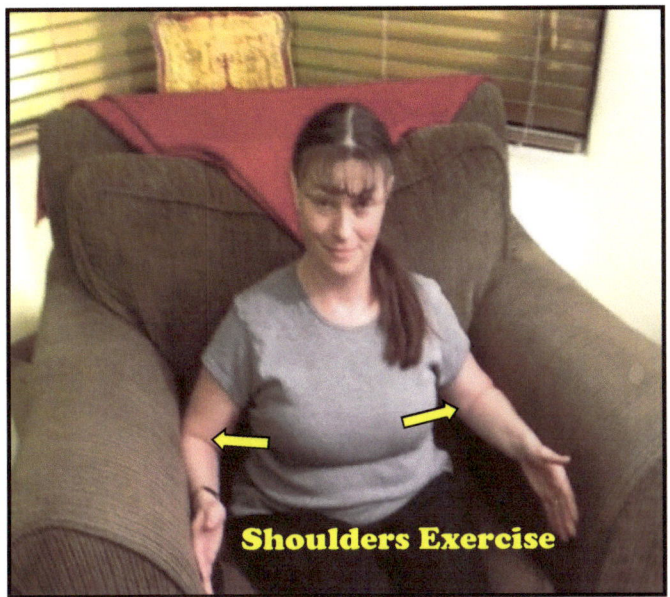

Shoulders Exercise

Press straight outward against the chair arms with both elbows. You guessed it … ten seconds … ten times.

It works muscles at the tops of your arms called the deltoid muscles. If you have a rotator cuff problem though, pass on this one.

Finally, let's go over the ones we all want most … the ***tummy muscles!***

# # #

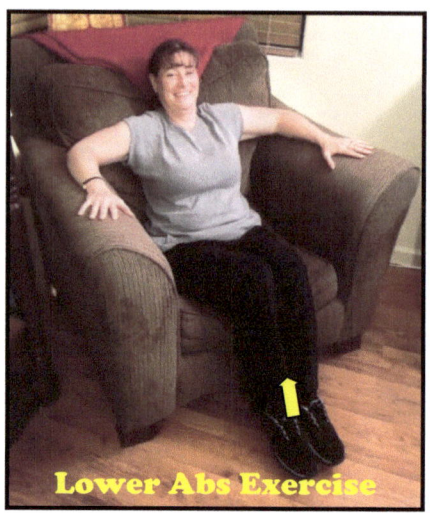

Lower Abs Exercise

Chapter Seven: The Abs!

I've always known that there's a "six-pack" in there on my tummy somewhere! The challenge is removing the padding on top of it so I can see it in the mirror!

I want to assure you that doing these exercises will help you develop muscle tone and burn more calories in your life. But I want to be realistic with you too. Even though you may be building those six pack abs, you may need to do other things to remove some of the padding on top of it ... like I do. I'll explain how to do this a bit later.

We'll work the abs in two different ways:

1) We'll work the lower abs first, and then

2) We'll work the upper abs.

But rest assured, we **_can_** do them slouching in the easychair!

Lower Abs Exercise: *Assume the position.* Slouch. Then lift your feet two inches off the floor and hold them. Do both of them at the same time. Feel the muscles in your lower tummy contracting.

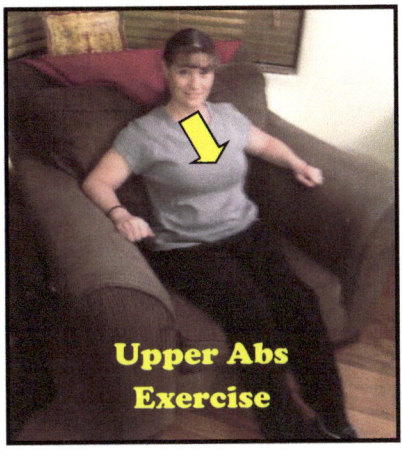

Your exertion is forward, as if you were going to get up.

Upper Abs Exercise

This will help work your upper quads too, but it's considered a lower abs (tummy) exercise.

This can require a considerable effort, so let's set some parameters for you. Lots of people have difficulty holding this position for a full 10 seconds. If you need to start with three seconds, or five seconds or seven seconds, that's quite all right. But set your first goal at ten seconds. Once you can hold for ten seconds, if you really want to trim down that tummy, slowly ease your way up to 15 or 20 seconds.

Do ten lifts in a set.

Upper Abs Exercise: Again, for this last exercise, *assume the position* one more time. Rest your hands on the chair arms. Let them go limp. Then raise your back and shoulders up and away from the seat back as if you were going to get out of the chair. But only come up three to four inches. Feel those tummy muscles getting tough and firm! Hold for ten seconds (if you can) and repeat ten times.

Now that you know what all of the exercises are, let's put them together in a regular program for you. It would be too inconvenient and uncomfortable to do them all, everyday!

February 2014

Sun	Mon	Tue	Wed	Thu	Fri	Sat
						1 Walk
2	3 Chair Workout	4 Walk	5 Chair Workout	6 Walk	7 Chair Workout	8 Walk
9	10 Chair Workout	11 Walk	12 Chair Workout	13 Chair Workout	14 ★Go out to dinner!	15 Walk
16	17 Chair Workout	18 Walk	19 Chair Workout	20 Walk	21 Chair Workout	22 Walk
23	24 Chair Workout	25 Walk	26 Chair Workout	27 Walk	28 Chair Workout Walk	

Chapter 8:
Developing Your Exercise Program

Building strength in muscles requires working them until they start to tire and then letting them rest and recover. We'll do this three different ways.

1) When you hold an exercise position for 10 seconds, follow it with a rest period of _two really deep breaths_ … in through your nose and out through your mouth. If you hold a position for 20 seconds, take a rest period of _three really deep breaths._ BREATHING prevents the soreness associated with exercise! It also promotes muscle health.

2) Rest for a full minute between **_sets._** For most of the exercises in this book, ten repetitions equals one set.

3) For most of the exercises, do three sets, one day a week. Do all three sets on the same day. (See chart on page 35.) For the abdominal exercises, however, do three sets on _each_ workout day. Abdominal exercises should be done more often than the other exercises to keep the muscles trim, slim and in great tone.

Doing the other exercises, only one day a week each, allows the body to create more mitochondria in between sessions to keep your energy levels up. It also gives tiny muscle fibers time to repair if necessary.   24

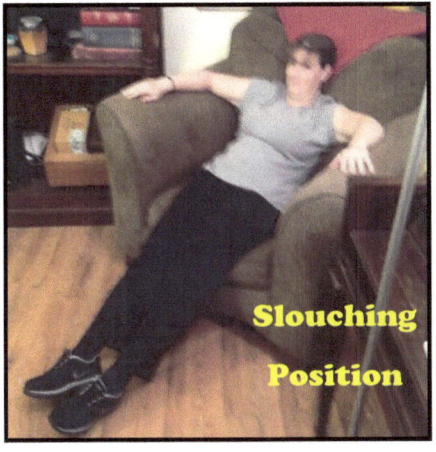

Slouching

Position

Pick three days out of the week to do your program. It may be Monday, Wednesday and Friday, for example. There should be at least one day between the days you choose.

Day One: On the first of your three exercise days, *do all five the Lower Extremity Exercises.*

After you've completed the Lower Extremity Exercises, do *both the Lower Abs* and *Upper Abs Exercises.*

Day Two: The middle day will require the most work. *Do all of the Torso Exercises.* Three of these are the chest exercises, so it's not as intense as it sounds.

When you complete all of the Torso Exercises, *do the Lower and Upper Ab Exercises again.*

Day Three: You get to take it easier on this day. Instead of five or more major exercises, there are only four. *Do the Neck and Upper back Exercises and follow these up with Lower and Upper Ab exercises too.*

Then take two days off and start over.

Keep in mind that this is the ideal schedule.

If a particular exercise hurts you DON'T DO IT. Skip it and go the next. Don't abandon the entire program because one exercise doesn't work out for you. Anything that you CAN do is going to help. The secret is to never give up.

There are four levels for doing these exercises. You can choose: **1) Cursory, 2) Beginner, 3) Intermediate or 4) The Full Exercise Program.**

1) **Cursory:** If you're in a hurry or you're out of shape and need to start easily and slowly, do the Cursory routine: Do each exercise only once and then go to the next. But do them with commitment and sincerity.

2) **Beginner:** Do one _set_ of each exercise for the day but with only _five_ repetitions in each set.

3) **Intermediate:** Do one _set_ of each exercise for the day with _ten to twenty_ repetitions in each set, depending on the exercise.

4) **The Full Exercise Program:** Do _three sets_ of ten repetitions for each exercise for the day.

You determine the level at which you're most comfortable. Balance that with what's giving you the best results.

# # #

Moving up from one level to the next: When do you know you're ready to kick it up a notch? Move up to "Beginner" from "Cursory" within the first 90 days _if you can_.

After that, your goal is to challenge yourself just a bit. You should feel a little tight after the workout, but pain is certainly not necessary. Ninety days at one level should prepare you for the next.

If moving up to the next level causes you too much discomfort, however, back off and try it again in another month.

If you can never feel comfortable with a next level, that's OK. Everybody's unique. There are no hard and fast rules. You make the decisions, but do try to challenge yourself when you can.

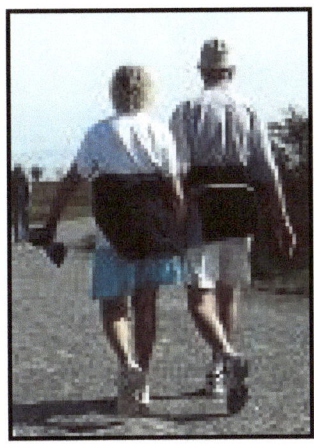

Chapter 9: Focus on Weight Loss ... Exercise

For all our efforts to strengthen muscles and get more fit, effective weight loss is more complex. There are actually no short cuts, regardless of all the pills, potions, diets, gadgets and other short cuts we read about and see advertised. You may be able to drop some weight with some of those things, but it will always be temporary.

Statistically, weight loss efforts with those short cuts nearly always results in regaining all of the weight lost plus an average of five pounds.

That's because they don't promote a permanent change in lifestyle.

This was one reason I wanted to create the Easychair Workout program. It's the easiest, most comfortable and least intrusive place from which to start a real change in *__lifestyle.__* After all, who wouldn't want to stay relaxed and comfy and work into exercise so easily?

Here's the thing about weight loss however. As much as we'd all like it to be something magic, it boils down to calories absorbed versus calories used *__in a limited time frame.__* If we absorb more calories than we burn during a period of a few hours, the body acts like a little

kid with a stash of candy. What it can't use now, *__it saves__*

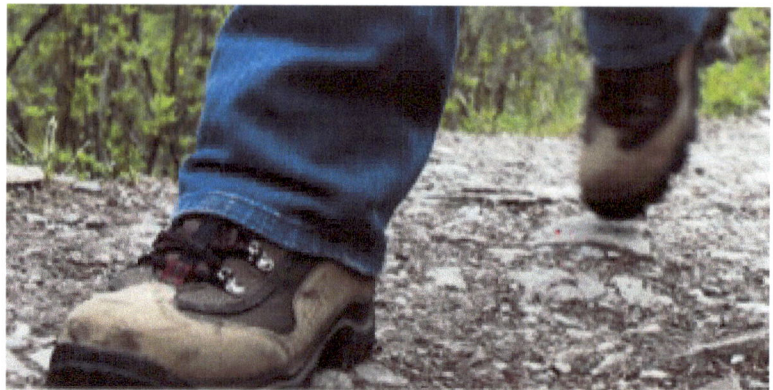

**for later.** The body saves calories by converting blood sugar to fat to burn for energy later.

The secret to burning that fat is to use more energy in the form of calories … _**in a short amount of time**_ … than we consume.

The greatest consumers of calories in the body are muscles … all of the muscles we've been talking about … plus the heart muscle.

Of the available exercises one could do on a regular basis, the benefits of walking appear to be right up near the top because walking works so many of those muscles … including the heart.

So if your ultimate goal for exercise is to lose weight, start by doing the Easychair Exercises. They'll give you more _**energy**_ on a regular basis. Then, when you have more energy 24/7/365, it's much easier to motivate yourself to do the more active fat-burning activities.

Try the Easychair Exercises for a month on a regular basis, then start your walking program to really burn off those calories quickly.

Start by walking to the end of your block and back or walking a couple hundred yards. Then add more distance each week until you're walking a mile at a time. Work up to a mile each way if time permits.

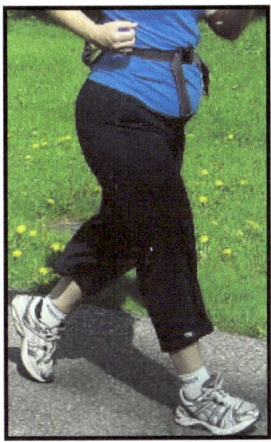

The best place to add your walking sessions to your exercise program is on the non-exercise days, on the days between your Easychair Exercises. So you'd be walking two to three times weekly.

When you walk, walk briskly enough to get your heart rate up to 120 beats per minute (30 beats every 15 seconds). Until you're in better shape, 120 should be plenty. Once you've kept your heart rate up to 120 beats a minute for 15 minutes, your body goes into a focused fat-burning mode.

That's your overall goal for walking to lose weight … keeping your heart rate over 120 longer than 15 minutes. For instance, if you're walking briskly for one hour, with your heart rate above 120, you'll be burning fat for a full 45 minutes!

Vigorous and ***continuous*** swimming can have similar results and add the trimming stimulus of the cold water. The cold requires burning more calories to keep you warm and stimulates your thyroid to be more active, increasing your metabolic rate.

# # #

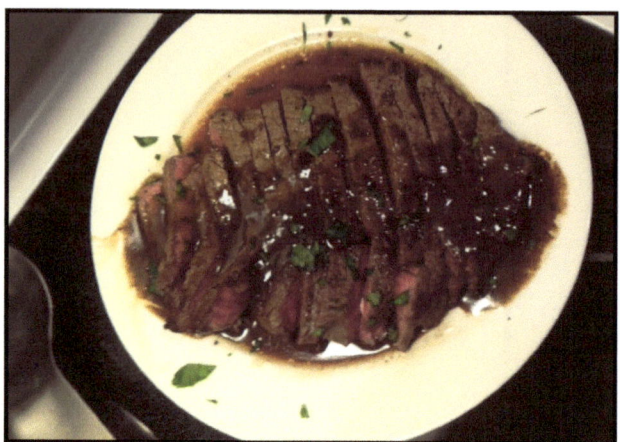

Chapter 10: Focus on Weight Loss ... Nutrition

In the previous chapter I briefly explained that accumulating fat is a matter of absorbing more calories ... ***in a limited amount of time*** ... than we can use.

Knowing some simple basics about food can help.

How much you eat is important ... true. But it's **_not_** the whole story.

How fast the calories end up in your cells to be used for energy is just as important. *If the calories aren't used in time, they're converted to fat.*

With that in mind, let's take a look at how fast different foods convert to useable calories.

There are only three basic nutrients—Proteins, Fats and Carbohydrates.

Proteins (meat, fish, poultry, hard cheeses, eggs) are made up of extremely long, convoluted, complicated molecules. They actually require the use of calories to break them down into their component parts to offer their own calories for use. It can take from 6 to 8 hours for that to happen.

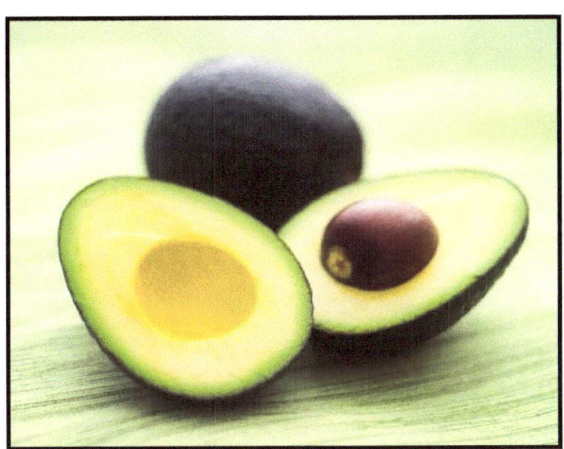

Therefore, eating protein provides calories and energy slowly … over an extended period of time. It offers your body the most amount of time to use the calories **_before_** your body has the opportunity to convert them to fat for later use.

Fats, including both animal fats and vegetable oils, are still pretty complicated, long-chain molecules. They hold 9 calories per gram compared to 4 calories per gram in carbohydrates. What the nutritionists DON'T tell us, however, is that some of those calories are burned to break down the fat; plus the process can take 3 to 5 hours to complete. So your body still has a good amount of time to use those calories as they become available, before your body can re-convert them into human fat. Plus fats turn off our hunger centers in the brain!

*By the way, the fat that ends up on our thighs, tummy and arms is **NEVER** the fat that we eat! Our immune systems would attack it and that would kill us. The fat on our bodies is always ... 100% of the time ... fat that <u>our own bodies make</u>. (Just FYI. It's a pet peeve of mine.)*

One of the reasons nutritionists vilify fats is because of their relationship to triglycerides, which are the building blocks that become cholesterol.

In order to build a triglyceride molecule, we need fat. But we also need carbohydrates. You can't build a triglyceride without **_both_**

HC3 ⌇ CH3

CH3   CH3

CH3

HO

Cholesterol

components.

It seems to be beyond the conception of grain-loving nutritionists that anybody could possibly restrict their carbohydrate intake, so they automatically attack fat by default.

The truth is, you can control your triglycerides … and therefore your cholesterol … by restricting your ***carbohydrates*** more easily than by restricting your fats.

Why?

Because carbohydrates stimulate insulin and insulin promotes cholesterol formation … LDL's … the "bad" ones. Fats aren't known to do that. So use heavy cream in your coffee and fry your eggs in butter, but pass on the toast, cinnamon rolls and pancakes.

Carbohydrates: Which brings us to the last of the three nutrients … carbohydrates. These are very simple molecules. The simplest ones are the sugars. The simplest of all is glucose … what your body sees as blood sugar … what your mitochondria convert to energy.

But they also include the "complex carbs" that the nutritionists want to promote as harmless and healthy.

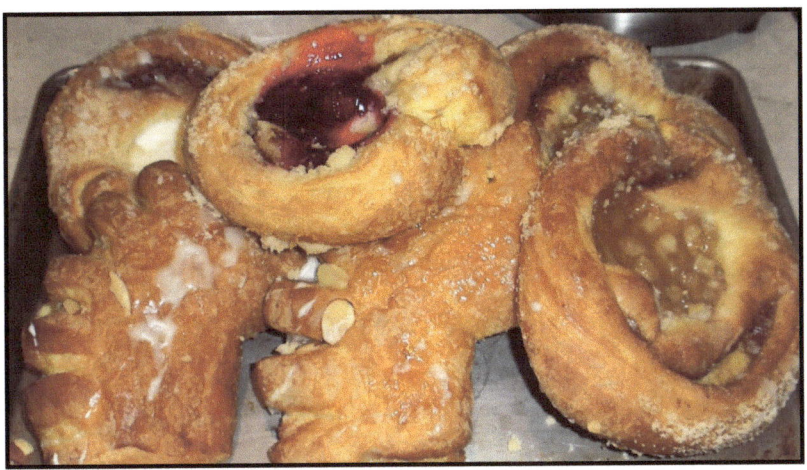

If your blood sugar consistently reads 90 to 100, two hours after you've eaten them, complex carbs may be tolerable for you. They're always better than simple carbs (sugars and starches). But if you have ANY blood sugar issues, even the complex carbs represent a threat to your waistline ... and your diabetic risks.

Weight-wise here's the issue. Because carbohydrates are such simple molecules, they break down _**very fast**_. Amylase enzymes in our saliva starts breaking them down as soon as you start chewing them! That's why they have such a great reputation for quick energy. "Quick" is the operative word here. They're completely digested in 30 minutes to two hours. If you haven't _**used**_ that energy in that short amount of time, your body "saves" it ... it converts it to FAT! Because of the TIME factor, _carbohydrates are converted to fat even more effectively than fats_!

Nutritionally then, to help drop weight, keep your carbohydrate intake to less than 100 grams per day. Avoid sugar, syrups, jams, jellies, rice, bread (including all things made with wheat and whole wheat) and potatoes.

Don't over-do on the fats but do enjoy them. And include at least 5 to 10 ounces of protein in your daily diet.

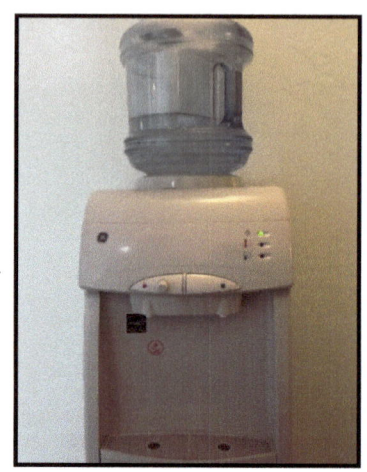

Also make sure to get enough water for good heart, kidney and joint health by dividing your weight in half and setting that number as your goal for ounces of water daily.

Incidentally, I've seen patients drop up to 40 pounds by just getting enough water and making no other changes in their lives! So this is a vital part of any effective weight loss program.

# # #

A 7-day Chart for Exercises, Walking and Rest

Easychair Exercises							
Exercises	Day 1	Off day	Day 2	Off day	Day 3	Off day	Off day
Quads Exercise	X						
Hamstrings Exercise	X						
Outer Thighs Exercise	X						
Inner Thighs Exercise	X						
Calves Exercise	X						
Low Back Exercise			X				
Love Handles Exercise			X				
Push Back Exercise			X				
Press Down Exercise			X				
Chest Exercise 1			X				
Chest Exercise 2			X				
Chest Exercise 3			X				
Neck Exercise					X		
Triceps Exercise					X		
Biceps Exercise					X		
Shoulder Exercise					X		
Lower Abs Exercise	X		X		X		
Upper Abs Exercise	X		X		X		
Walking		X		X		X	

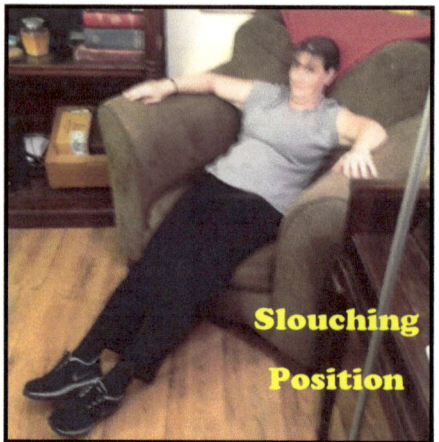

Slouching Position

Summary

This book is small, but powerful!

It's written for people, like me, who are reluctant to get out of that easychair to start getting in shape.

But we all know we have to be in good physical shape to be as healthy as we can be and to live our lives to the fullest.

Sit there. Be lazy. But get in shape anyway. You're going to be **_SOOO_** glad you did this!

If you would like for Dr. Boatright to speak to your group about the Easychair Workout, or about training your people to supervise the Easychair Workout, please contact him at ralby@frontiernet.net.

Also ask us about our _"I work Out in My Easychair"_ tee shirts, sweat shirts and jackets.

And watch for our upcoming video.

Yours for awesome health,

Dr. Rick Boatright

Other Books by Dr. Rick Boatright

"Surviving Type II Diabetes" … Amazon .com

"Surviving Type II Diabetes, Second Edition" … Kindle

"Crossing the Veil" … Kindle

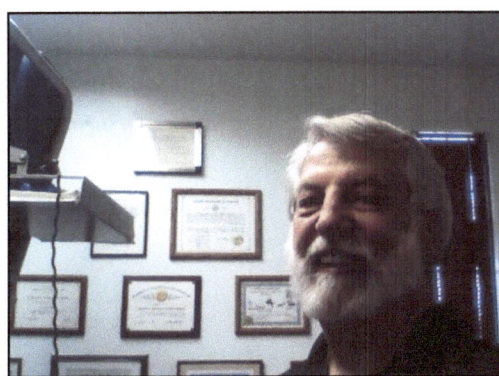

About the author:

Dr. Rick Boatright has been a doctor of chiropractic since the 1980's. He's a world-recognized expert with gentle, instrument approaches to chiropractic.

Dr. Boatright received a certification to work with animals in 1998. He works quite often with dogs and horses.

In 2006, he earned a certification as a Golf Injury Specialist.

His great love, however, is writing. "The word 'doctor' means teacher," he says, "and I take that seriously. Writing offers one of the best ways to accomplish that."

To contact Dr. Boatright, e-mail him at ralby@frontiernet.net. To avoid the computer interpreting it as spam, in the subject line, type "about docs chair."

See his practice web site at **www.drrickboatright.com.**

See his writing web site at **www.readem.net.**

And if you will, please tell a friend or loved one about the **Easychair Workout.** You just might save a life!

The Complete Easychair Workout Program   **Dr. Rick Boatright**

Notes:

The Complete Easychair Workout Program   Dr. Rick Boatright

Notes:

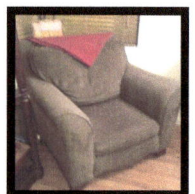

Dr. Rick Boatright
P. O. Box 3330,
Pinetop, AZ 85935-3330

www.ingramcontent.com/pod-product-compliance
Lightning Source LLC
Chambersburg PA
CBHW050755290526
45792CB00008B/2198